READY,
Set,
shrink!

Lori Ferrante

ISBN: 1-4392-2266-5
ISBN-13: 9781439222669

Visit www.booksurge.com to order additional copies.

Dedication

To my parents for their unconditional love, support, and guidance throughout this process and in everything I have ever done! You've helped me realize how important it is to never sit it out when I could choose to dance instead! I love you!

To my in-laws who have always trusted in me, even though they may have had doubts about my decisions.

To my children (Ariana, Chiara, and Jack) who always encouraged me to "keep shrinking" and were always waiting until I "lost" them (as in forty pounds equaled how much my son weighed at the time)—I've now "lost" each one of them!

To Cindy, Deb, and Janet for being the best friends a girl could have.

To the support group at St. Elizabeth's Medical Center (especially Anne) a huge thanks for being there for me, always answering my questions (no matter how blunt or personal), and for helping me get through it all!

To Dr. Nicole Pecquex who always did the best thing for me, even when I tried to convince her otherwise! You gave me back to the world with your gifts.

And lastly, to my husband, John, who, despite his initial reservations, tells everyone who will listen how proud he is of me and how fabulous I have done (not to mention how great I look)!

Without each and every one of you, I could not have done so well!

Love,
Lori

Table of Contents

Chapter 1:Why You Need This Book   1

GET READY

Chapter 2:Pre-Testing & Other Necessary Evils   3
Chapter 3:Preparing For Surgery   5
Chapter 4:Nutrition Basics   11

GET SET

Chapter 5:Dumping & Other "Fun" Activities   15
Chapter 6:Feeling Stuffed on Liquids (Stages 1-3)   19
Chapter 7:The Joy of Chewing (Stage 4)   23
Chapter 8:Back to REAL Food (Stage 5)   27
Chapter 9:Supplements Galore   29

SHRINK

Chapter 10:Back to Reality   31
Chapter 11:Unexpected Weight Loss Issues   35
Chapter 12:New Treats   39
Chapter 13:Plastic Surgery & Beyond   43
Chapter 14:Then There's You   47

Appendices

Pre-Surgery Shopping List   A-1   49
Body Measurements   A-2   51
Daily Tracking Sheet (Stage 3)   A-3   53

Daily Tracking Sheet (Stage 4)   A-4   55
Daily Tracking Sheet (Stage 5)   A-5   57
Sugars   A-6   59
Protein Sources   A-7   61

1.Why You Need This Book

"After Gastric Bypass Surgery (GBS), you will need to take about forty minutes to eat four ounces of food." Are they kidding?! Most people today don't spend forty minutes eating in an entire day, let alone one meal! This book is about helping men and women to merge their "real" lives with their post-GBS requirements.

Before deciding to have GBS, I read many books on the pros and cons of the various bariatric surgery methods as well as stories of patients who did well (and some who did not). All these books were very useful in the decision-making process. Nothing, however, really prepared me for life afterward.

On August 28, 2006, I reported for my GBS weighing 267 pounds at five feet two inches tall and thirty-nine years old. When I woke up in the recovery room, the real fun began! I spent countless hours on the computer surfing the Internet trying to find answers to my questions—the "non-medical" kind that my doctors couldn't really answer as they had never actually been through the experience.

I found over forty books on the subject of "gastric bypass surgery." Most of them were the ones I had read **before** my surgery. The books that had to do with **after** the surgery were mostly cookbooks! This was NOT what I was looking for! Where were the books that could help me now, in my post-op day-to-day struggles? Nowhere, that's where! UNTIL NOW!!!!

I'm not a doctor, nurse, nutritionist, or psychiatrist, but I am someone who has lived through it and done very well! This book is based on my journey, but its intent is to share with you some of the methods I used to help make the transition from my life "before the surgery" to the "new me" after. It's all of my personal experiences and research, consolidated into checklists, helpful hints, shopping lists, and more.

Today's busy men and women need convenience, fast results, and quick lists to move them back into the mainstream of their busy lives without a lot of fanfare. Whether you're a corporate executive, a school crossing guard, a homemaker, self-employed, or retired, your life is complex and you want easy answers that work in the real world—not just on paper. This book is about helping you find ways to merge your "real world" with your new "post-op GBS world." This won't always be easy and sometimes it might even seem down-right impossible. But with enough planning and guidance, it can be fairly simple if you know the tips before you go into surgery.

READY, Set, shrink!!!!!!!!!!

2.Pre-Testing & Other Necessary Evils

You finally make the difficult decision to have gastric bypass surgery (GBS) and then you discover the medical world of "hurry up and wait"! You will most likely have to undergo months of testing to make sure you qualify for the surgery and that you are physically and mentally ready for it. These tests are *necessary evils*, but they are actually very important. All of this pre-testing is an effort to minimize potential complications that could arise and endanger your health and life if they were left undiscovered. So, grin and bear it—it's in your best interest.

Weight loss: Most programs will require you to lose a certain amount of weight before performing GBS. In my case it was five percent of my weight, which was about twelve to fifteen pounds. The purpose of the weight loss is to shrink the liver and make surgery technically easier.

Gallbladder ultrasound: The purpose of this test is to make sure your gallbladder is healthy and that you don't have gallstones. If there's a problem, they may choose to remove your gallbladder before proceeding with GBS.

Cardiac evaluation: This could be as simple as an EKG or much more involved depending on what is discovered. If any problems are determined, then your road to GBS hits a roadblock because your heart issues need to be resolved and/or stabilized before proceeding (which could take months, but hopefully not).

Sleep study: Most men and women over two hundred-fifty pounds (which is everyone who's considering GBS) have some form of sleep apnea. This is a condition that interrupts breathing during sleep. This painless test requires you to sleep overnight at either a hospital or sleep facility. You arrive about one hour before your normal bedtime and you go to sleep while they study you (with wires stuck to your face, nose, etc.). Any findings require treatment before GBS. If you are found to have sleep apnea, there's a delay as you arrange for a special device called a CPAP (continuous positive airway pressure) machine to assist your breathing. This machine is used during sleep and it can take some getting used to. Sometimes patients have to try several different machines before they find the one that works best for them.

Blood work: Fairly routine, but lots of blood will be taken to make sure that all bodily functions are normal. Again, any abnormalities need to be resolved before proceeding with GBS.

Pulmonary function test (PFT): Most obese people have some type of breathing problem and these issues need to be investigated and treated prior to undergoing GBS.

Psychiatric evaluation: You have to meet with one or more psychiatrists so they can determine your "emotional fitness" for GBS. The doctors want to make sure that you understand the ramifications of what you are about to do and that you are willing to make all the necessary changes that are required for success. If you are unsure about doing this surgery in any way at all, DO NOT DO IT! You need to be 400 percent committed to doing this! This should NEVER be done half-heartedly, but rather with gusto!

3.Preparing For Surgery

If you get nothing else out of my book, I hope you remember that the most important thing is to PLAN AHEAD! Your body is going to be going through a complete overhaul (and your mental state too), so you need to make your first few post-op weeks as easy as possible. There are lots of items that I found I needed AFTER I got home from the hospital and had to rely on others to get for me. Here are the things I would recommend you get (or do) BEFORE you go in for surgery:

Protein shakes: You will need to have at least two cans of this stuff (seventy grams of protein) a day and it's not easy to find. You can go to Vitamin Shoppe (or online at www.vitaminshoppe.com) or Trader Joe's (or a similar store near you). Buy one can of each flavor they carry that's high protein and no sugar added (using Splenda or a similar substitute is fine). Take them home and try them out. Some taste really bad and you won't be able to tolerate them, but eventually you'll find one you like (and hopefully more than one flavor).

Then you need to buy a couple of cases of them to have on hand, waiting for when you get home from the hospital. You will be drinking this and other liquids exclusively for about ten to fourteen days depending on your program. Plus, after you progress to ground foods, you will still supplement with one can or so a day until you get back to all solid foods. I still keep some around because when I get sick (like with the flu), sometimes it's the only way I know I'll get my protein in!

GladWare "mini round" containers (½ cup size): The first several months, your new stomach size can only hold four ounces at a time. I would open up several cans of protein shakes and pour them into these small containers, put the lids on, and store them in the fridge. The top shelf of my fridge was reserved for my foods. At any given point, I could look in and see about twenty different containers of different colored drinks. It made life so much easier to just grab one of those containers, knowing it was exactly the right portion size, pop the top, and go!

Later on in the food stages, I would use them for ground beef or tuna salad, or whatever was on the menu. All were pre-measured and I didn't have to think about it after I made them and put them away. Whenever I had ten to fifteen minutes, I would set up additional containers so when life got busy (as everyone's does), I did not have trouble staying with it.

Food scale: You need to get a small kitchen scale to weigh your food. Remember, for the first several months your stomach will only hold about four ounces at a time, so a scale that goes up to one pound is more than sufficient. For the first year, I continued to weigh all my food when I was home. It really helps you learn to judge what a "real size" portion is for when you go out and don't have your scale or small containers with you.

Food processor: A small food chopper or processor will be helpful during Stage 4 (weeks three and four after surgery) as all foods need to be ground or pureed.

Pill crusher: For the first couple of months, every pill you take will have to be crushed. I went through all the crushers they sell at the pharmacy counters and gave up because the powder kept getting stuck in the little grooves (or I wasn't strong enough to turn the top to make it work)! I ended up with a nice, old-fashioned marble mortise and pestle that was actually bought at a kitchen store (designed for crushing herbs). Best $12 I ever spent!

Powdered drink mixes or flavored waters: I hate the taste of water and Crystal Light, and Fruit$_2$O made getting my liquids in each day a LOT easier! Fruit$_2$O is great because it's a pre-mixed, non-carbonated water with fruit flavoring and no added sugars. If you don't like the flavored waters, you can buy a multi-pack of bottled water with the sport tops on them and then add the Crystal Light. This way you can have something that tastes good (without added sugars) and still meet your liquid requirement each day. Reuse the bottles until you can't anymore. To this day I have two of them in my refrigerator at all times mixed up and ready to go when I head out the door. The portable "on the go" size packets of Crystal Light are great to take on vacation or to put in your car too.

Surgical recovery items: When you get home from the hospital, your stomach muscles will be completely shot and getting into or out of bed (or even lying flat) can be a big problem. If you have a recliner chair (or can borrow one from a friend), it's the best place to sleep for the first week or two. Also, make sure you have enough gauze pads and first aid tape handy to change the dressings on your incisions.

Body measurements: Take your measurements the day (or week) before your surgery. Every month thereafter, take them again. You will be amazed at the changes happening all over your body. It's a real pick-me-up. I recommend you measure all of the following: neck, bust, waist, hips, thigh, calf, ankle, upper arm, forearm, wrist, shoe size (including width), and ring size. There are going to be months along the way when you won't lose any pounds, but you will continue to lose inches. Keeping these measurements will be the most amazing motivational tool you have.

	Pre-Op	6 wks.	2 mths.	3 mths.	4 mths.	5 mths.	6 mths.
Weight	267	232	221	216	202	194	190
Wrist	7.5	7.25	7.0	7.0	6.75	6.75	6.5
Forearm	12.5	11.75	11.25	11.0	10.75	10.75	10.5
Upper Arm	18.5	16.0	15.5	15.5	15.0	15.0	15.0
Neck	16.0	15.0	14.75	14.25	14.25	13.75	13.5
Bust	48.0	44.5	44.0	43.0	42.0	41.5	40.5
Waist	45.0	43.0	41.5	40.0	37.5	37.0	36.5
Hips	58.0	55.0	52.5	51.0	50.0	49.5	47.0
Thigh	27.0	25.5	24.5	24.0	23.0	22.5	22.0
Calf	18.5	17.5	17.0	17.0	16.5	16.25	16.0
Ankle	10.5	10.0	10.0	10.0	9.75	9.75	9.5
Ring Size	9.0	8.5	8.0	7.0	6.5	6.0	6.0
Shoe Size	8ww	8ww	8w	8w	8w	8w	8m

Bathing suit photos: I know you're sitting there saying, "No way am I getting into a bathing suit and having someone take my photo!" Trust me on this one. We do not see ourselves as we really are and that photo will be the one true measure of what you looked like (and how others saw you) before this journey. Make sure you stand next to something stationary (in my case it was a fence) so you can repeat the photo later to see the difference. A picture really is worth a thousand words!

Daily Tracking Sheet (DTS): I created a form that helped me track how much protein and liquids I had daily and to make sure I took all my medicines and supplements. With all the things going on that you have to keep track of, having a checklist made it easier to make sure I was on target at all times. As I progressed from liquids to ground/pureed and then to solids, I changed the form to suit that week's needs. Every Sunday I printed out a new one with new dates and added new foods to the list as I expanded my repertoire. To this day I still use the chart at least once or twice a month to make sure I'm getting all my proteins and liquids in (and not just assuming I am). Here's a sample of my DTS for a Stage 3 week:

Item	SUN 9/3	MON 9/4	TUE 9/5	WED 9/6	THU 9/7	FRI 9/8	SAT 9/9
Zantac (am)							
Thyroid (am)							
Atenolol (am)							
Protein shake (4 oz.=12 g.)							
Protein shake (4 oz.=12 g.)							
Protein shake (4 oz.=12 g.)							
Protein shake (4 oz.=12 g.)							
Protein shake (4 oz.=12 g.)							
Protein shake (4 oz.=12 g.)							
Fage yogurt (3.5 oz.=9 g.)							
Fage yogurt (3.5 oz.=9 g.)							
Fage yogurt (3.5 oz.=9 g.)							
Cream of rice cereal (4 oz.=2 g.)							
Fruit$_2$O-16 oz							
Fruit$_2$O-16 oz							
Multivitamin							
Atenolol (pm)							
PROTEIN (70 g.= target)							
LIQUIDS (32 oz.= min.)							

Sugar-free medicines: You need to stock up on at least one container of sugar-free cough syrup and some Tylenol (their "Go Tabs" aren't bad and are actually chewables without sugar). Nothing worse than getting a sore throat or cough a few weeks after surgery and realizing you can't take the good old Nyquil or Robitussin you have in the medicine cabinet because it's all sugar, which can cause "dumping" (see Chapter 5).

Multivitamins: I highly recommend that you go for a children's sugar-free chewable to start. One-A-Day Bugs Bunny and Scooby Doo have more than adequate vitamins for your needs. If you've ever tasted an adult multivitamin crushed up, you'll appreciate the kids' sugar-free instead! No gagging required! Remember, it'll be two to three months before you'll be able to swallow pills whole, and vitamin supplements are usually larger than most other pills.

MedicAlert emblem: One of the "horror" stories I had heard before my surgery was that some woman was in an accident and went to an emergency room and no one knew she had had GBS. For some medical reason, they decided to put a tube down her throat. In doing this, they inadvertently punctured her new small pouch (as it's no longer in exactly the same place or size as it should be) causing problems that lead to her death! This could have been avoided if she had been able to tell them about her GBS or been wearing a MedicAlert emblem. I was so freaked out that I could be in some kind of accident or something and not be able to tell anyone about my GBS, so I signed up for a MedicAlert bracelet and wear it at all times (www.medicalert.com or 800-432-5378). It is engraved with "GBS, no NSAIDS, no NG tube w/out scope."

Firstly, it tells doctors that you had GBS, so your stomach and intestines are routed differently. The "no NSAIDS" means that you should not be given any anti-inflammatory drugs (NSAIDS) such as aspirin or Motrin. The last part means that they should not place any naso-gastric (NG) tubes down your throat without using an endoscopic camera to visually guide them (so they don't puncture anything)! It gives me a level of comfort and security knowing that if I can't speak for myself, my MedicAlert emblem will. The $50-$100 it will cost to enroll you in the program and get an emblem of some sort to wear is cheap compared to the value of your life!

NOTES

4.Nutrition Basics

Basically, GBS works by reducing the size of your stomach from about the size of a football to the size of a golf ball. This new smaller stomach pouch limits how much and what kinds of foods you can eat. Therefore, you eat a lot less calories and lose lots of weight. A portion of your small intestine is also "bypassed," so your ability to digest and absorb certain foods is impaired (called "malabsorption") as a result. You may no longer be able to eat sugary or fatty foods. But that's okay because this helps weight loss.

Remember, this surgery is not a quick, easy fix for obesity. It is a complete and total overhaul of your digestive system and your whole world. It can be an amazing thing if you take it seriously, but if you don't, it's just like all the other diets you've tried and failed, except with more long-term, serious health consequences.

The first few months after surgery, your meals should be no more than four ounces (½ cup) in size and should take forty to sixty minutes to eat. Over the first year or so, your stomach will gradually stretch so you can eat more food, but the portions should still remain small. A year after surgery and forever, try not to exceed more than eight ounces (one cup) per meal. This will help to maintain your weight loss. You will also need to separate your eating and drinking and learn to stop when you *first* feel full.

The basic nutritional plan for eating after your surgery is:

Stage 1 (24 hours after surgery) – Colored water: The first thing you are given is water with a dye in it (in my case it was blue). This is done so the doctors can make sure there are no leaks in your new stomach pouch and surgical sites that could cause infections.

Stage 2 (24-48 hours after surgery) – Clear sugar-free liquids: Things like broth, gelatin, popsicles, and juices. Should be in four-ounce portions and take ten minutes or so to drink each ounce.

Stage 3 (Days 3-14) – Sugar-free liquids: This means adding yogurt, pudding, milk, protein shakes, and things of that nature. Again, four-ounce servings should take about forty minutes to consume. Eggs are also part of this group, but most patients I have spoken to had a really hard time digesting eggs for three to six months, so don't be surprised if you have difficulty too.

Stage 4 (Weeks 3 & 4) – Ground/Pureed foods: Ground meats, cottage cheese, applesauce, oatmeal, etc. (still no added sugars) plus all the other previous stage foods.

Stage 5 (Weeks 5+) – Solid foods: Start out slowly by adding one new food a day (cut very small and chewed completely). By week 7 or 8, you will be back to all real, normal foods. Be aware, however, that some people can take up to six months to get back to solid food.

There are about five key things to always remember: ***protein first***; no added sugars (not even a little); frequent small meals; always drink your required liquids; and exercise. If you can stick to these unwritten "rules," you will be a lot better off than those who don't.

Protein is important because it helps you lose weight healthfully and to have the best surgical outcome. Most programs want you to have fifty to seventy grams of protein a day, which sounds daunting at best! However, if you consider that one of those protein shakes has about thirty-five grams per can, that's only two cans a day (which also just about meets your thirty-two ounces of liquids too)!

When you are back to solid foods, it actually is pretty easy to reach your protein target every day. For instance, one ounce of chicken has seven grams of protein. So if you eat a typical four-ounce serving of chicken at lunch that is twenty-eight grams of protein. Then you will have more protein at dinner. You probably also had some at breakfast (an egg has seven grams of protein). You can see how easy it is to get that protein in if you plan ahead and remember the "protein first" rule.

Whatever program you are following should have a nutritionist who will help you with the specific types of foods you can eat within each "stage" of the process. You also need to meet with this person several times in the first month or two after surgery to make sure that you are discussing any problems you may be having. Don't be afraid to call (or e-mail if they're so inclined) this person if you have any questions about your nutrition. Getting all the required protein, liquids, and supplements is vital to successful weight loss and overall health!

Other things to remember during the first few months are:

- eat and drink small portions very slowly;
- don't have any added sugars (see Chapter 5 for complete list);
- no carbonated beverages;
- no drinking straws;
- no chewing gum or sucking on hard candy;
- separate your liquids from your solids;
- keep a daily food diary (see Daily Tracking Sheet in Chapter 3);
- avoid carbohydrates (bread, crackers, pasta, etc.);
- avoid fatty and fried foods (pizza, fried chicken, etc.);
- choose fat-free dairy products instead of higher fat options; and
- stop eating at the first sign of fullness.

As the months progress, these restrictions will lighten up somewhat, but always consult with your nutritionist before making any changes or adjustments to your diet.

NOTES

5.Dumping & Other "Fun" Activities

Dumping: With your newly routed digestive process, if you consume sugars, they move very quickly from the stomach to the small intestine. This "dumping" of sugars causes your system to be very unhappy and it rebels by giving you feelings of nausea, abdominal cramps, sweating or hot flashes, and (ultimately) diarrhea. The sugars that are usually acceptable are: fructose, aspartame, lactose, sucralose, Splenda, Equal, Nutra-Sweet, and saccharin. Not acceptable added sugars are: sucrose, sugar, brown sugar, turbinado sugar, high-fructose corn syrup, corn syrup, honey, maple syrup, pure/organic cane sugar, confectioner's sugar, and molasses (see Appendix A-6).

I made the mistake of buying a liquid multivitamin so I wouldn't have to worry about the crushing. However, I did not read the label carefully and failed to notice that the number one ingredient was corn syrup. I drank the required one tablespoon dose of the vitamin. Within thirty minutes, I experienced the most painful gas bubble-type pains I ever experienced in my life (times ten)! I was flushed, felt nauseous, and doubled over from the gas pains. This went on for FIVE hours! When the gas worked its way out (by moving to the final phase—diarrhea) I was thrilled because it meant the end of the dumping. Trust me, once you experience this, you will NOT want it to happen again!

I began reading every label of every food before I put it in my body. There was not enough money in the world to make me eat something again with sugar in it if that was what I was going to experience! It certainly helps to keep you on the straight and narrow about sugar! And I wasn't even doing anything "bad"—just taking my vitamin! UGH! Not a pleasant experience! Fortunately, if you stay away from sugar (make sure to read your labels), this will not happen to you! It is completely avoidable! Now, some people are fortunate not to experience this side effect, but take it from me, it's better not to know if it will affect you or not. Avoid it at all costs!

Sticking/Vomiting: If you don't chew your food into small enough pieces and leave enough time in between bites, food tends to get "stuck" and sit at the opening to your new, smaller stomach. So then you think...if the food's not small enough to fit through, then the only place for it to go is back the way it came! Yup, you guessed it—you're going to have to throw it back up! A completely gross thought!

However, vomiting after GBS is so much less awful than before. You sort of gag a few times and up it comes. It's definitely not something you want to do often, but it's not the trauma that you envision. Don't let yourself get so worried about foods sticking that you don't try new things. Remember to chew a lot and go slowly, and most of the time you'll be fine. But I don't know a single person who didn't experience sticking at least once.

Nausea: Feels like a "gnawing feeling" in your stomach and can happen between meals when your stomach is empty. Eat a small amount of food (even a bite or two) and it will usually go away. Sometimes, if you're taking vitamins or other medicines on an empty stomach, that can do it too. Always take pills with some kind of food and make sure to space them out during the day (don't take them all at once).

Dehydration: Now that you can no longer "chug" liquids, you need to be careful to drink non-carbonated, decaffeinated, sugar-free liquids throughout the day. Gone are the days when you were working outside in the summer and would get hot and sweaty and then you'd drink a huge glass of lemonade. Now, with your smaller stomach, you can only take a few sips. Therefore, drinking small sips throughout the day (a few sips every thirty to forty-five minutes) will keep you hydrated.

Dehydration can cause a drop in your blood pressure, dizziness, and even fainting. Keep a water bottle with you at all times and keep taking sips. Easiest way for me was the plastic bottles with the pop-up tops so I didn't have to screw and unscrew a cap. Sounds lazy on my part, but it actually made it quicker and easier, which helped me stick to it.

Hiccups: Have you ever seen how babies are always hiccupping and you think to yourself, "that's so weird, what's that about?" Well, that will happen to you too! Basically, you are re-training your body how to eat and in the beginning few months, you hiccup a LOT as air gets trapped in your new smaller stomach. This is one of the reasons they don't want you to drink from straws or have anything carbonated—too much air to get trapped in that tiny pouch. It's not big, painful hiccups, just small, annoying ones. It lessens over the first few months until it no longer occurs for you more than anyone else. Just one of those "weird" things that happens, but be assured that it's all part of the process of re-educating your body about its new digestive tract.

Tummy gurgles: Any time I ate or drank anything at all, my stomach would start to gurgle (like a bathtub when it drains)! It's the weirdest thing! To this day, if I wait too long to eat between meals, when I do eat, my stomach gurgles for a good five to ten minutes as it's processing the food.

Flatulence: Lots of patients experience excess gas after GBS. Again, it's your body re-learning how to process food from the top to the bottom of the system (so to speak). It can be annoying and sometimes embarrassing, but it's all part of the process. Eventually it will lessen to a normal amount. Until then, just grin and bear it.

Hair loss: If you don't consume enough protein on a daily basis, it can lead to hair loss. The kind where you're shampooing your hair and when you pull your hands away from your lathering, you get clumps of hair along with that soap. This is a temporary situation and if you increase your protein intake, it will gradually lessen and return to normal. Another good reason to follow your nutritionist's guidelines!

Plateaus: No one ever told me that you can experience weeks or even months with no weight loss. I thought that was not possible with the extreme nature of this surgery, but it is. When I didn't lose any weight for over five weeks, I immediately began to worry and have self-doubt that I was going to be the one person in the world that this didn't work for. Not possible! Keep doing what you're doing and the weight will eventually drop. It's another good time to look at your body measurements and you will see progress there if not on the scale.

Intoxication: Since your body now absorbs everything you put into your mouth differently, one thing that will probably change is the way your body reacts to alcohol. Most GBS patients absorb alcohol much more quickly into their bodies. There have been reports of GBS patients who went out with friends, drank one glass of wine, and were pulled over on the way home by police for driving under the influence (and blowing the legal limits on a breathalyzer).

The crazy thing is that sometimes you can have one or two drinks and be fine, and another time, a half glass will make you black out and get completely loopy. So it's better to stick close to home when you're drinking or make sure you have a designated driver.

6.Feeling Stuffed On Liquids (Stages 1-3)

How hard can it be, you think, to drink thirty-two ounces of liquids a day?! Right?! Wrong!!! And, oh, by the way, you also have to have fifty to seventy grams of protein too! It's very tough when you have no appetite at all and a few sips make you feel completely stuffed (like you used to after eating Thanksgiving dinner with all the trimmings). And to top it all off, the protein shakes that are available taste less than spectacular (it's not exactly a yummy Friendly Fribble)!

Protein drinks tend to taste better if you drink them when they're ice cold. What I did was get out a bunch of my GladWare half-cup mini rounds and pour the shakes into these cups. I put the lids on them and stored them in the refrigerator for me to have throughout the week. When it's time for a shake, you just grab one of the cups, take the top off, and drink. No measuring at that point.

It was also easy to keep track because, for me, I knew I had to drink six of those little cups each day to reach my seventy grams of protein and thirty-two ounces of liquids. It's also easy to grab a couple of them if you're heading off to work or running errands. No guessing if you've had enough (don't want to stretch that stomach pouch) and no half-empty cans left sitting around in the refrigerator (ready to get knocked over)!

On top of the protein shakes, you still need to have other "liquids." Yogurt is a great protein source that also counts as a liquid (which in those early days is important to get the most bang for your swallowing buck)! The problem with most yogurts on the market is that they only have about five grams of protein per serving.

Fortunately, there is, in my opinion, an amazing yogurt called "Fage 0%" which is a Greek-style yogurt that has thirteen grams of protein (almost three times as much as a typical yogurt). It only comes in "plain" flavor (which I was not wild about), but I found that if I added one packet of Splenda to the 5.3 oz. container and mixed it in, it tasted more like vanilla and was actually really yummy! I, again, would open a couple of those containers, mix in the Splenda, and then separate it into my little half-cup GladWare containers. And then when it was time to eat, I would grab one of my cups and know it was the exact size I should be having and I didn't have to think about measuring or mixing at that point.

I found that very few places carry Fage and those that did were often out of it. Whole Foods carries the full line, but not everyone has those stores in their area. If you go to their website (www.fageusa.com) there is a section that tells you which stores sell it. Another company called Chobani (www.chobani.com) also sells a non-fat, plain Greek yogurt that has been popping up lately in more mainstream grocery stores. Later on as you progress to solid foods, you can also add a tablespoon of Smuckers "no sugar added" jam and turn it into other flavors (like strawberry or apricot).

The rest of the liquids were made up of broths, sugar-free Jell-O, and Crystal Light. It's not easy to get all the liquids in that they want you to (my program wanted a minimum of thirty-two ounces). You need to pace yourself and start early each day. You can't get to noontime and realize that because you're not hungry you haven't had anything yet to "eat" and then try to squeeze it all in the next six hours. It won't work. Your stomach is too small and can't handle so much in such a short period of time. That's why the Daily Tracking Sheet (see Appendices) is so helpful. If you check off each thing as you eat or drink it, it keeps you on target to meet your protein and liquid goals each day. The more you stick to those goals, the better your weight loss will be and the healthier you will feel.

The doctors don't make up these numbers just to make you crazy (though sometimes I thought they did)! There are real scientific reasons behind it, and you need to do your best to meet these goals every day. This is not something that should be taken lightly. You need to do as the doctors tell you or this will not work. As you progress to more solid foods, it becomes easier. But in the liquid stage, stick with the protein shakes and the Fage yogurt (if you can find it) and you should be fine.

NOTES

7.The Joy of Chewing (Stage 4)

Ah, to chew food again! Even if it is ground turkey, chicken, pork, or beef (which all tastes the same after being cooked), it's better than days on end of liquids! It's kind of scary when you think about it, but a huge step forward. I remember how excited I was to be able to actually bite into something after fourteen days of only liquids. Then you start to experience the problems. As a mom of three young children, I'm used to not eating my food hot all at once because I'm always interrupted. But for those of you who are used to your food being hot on your plate from beginning to end, this is going to be a bigger challenge.

This takes me back to my little half-cup GladWare containers. For example, I would cook up a package of ground chicken, add my flavorings and spices, and then take out my scale and containers. I would weigh each one out so there was four ounces in each, put the covers on, and store them in the refrigerator. Then when it was time to eat, I'd take out one small container, throw it in the microwave for thirty seconds, grab a spoon, and I was ready to go.

If you work outside the home, this is easy too because you can put two or more containers in a lunch bag (or briefcase) with some plastic spoons and you're set for the day. No worrying about how you're going to get the foods in while at work. Until you're back on all solid foods, there's no way you can avoid being "different" from everyone around you. So accept that, remember that you are doing this to improve your health, and ignore those who are less than charitable toward your situation.

By the time the ground/pureed stage is over, you are VERY glad because it gets really boring. The flavors available to you at this point are not the most exciting, but it's temporary. Keep your eyes on the goal and you'll make it through. Below are a couple of really simple recipes that will help make ground meat a little less boring:

Peach/Mango Chicken:

1 lb. ground chicken
3-3.9 oz. containers of Mott's "no sugar added" Peach Medley applesauce

1. Brown ground chicken in skillet
2. Drain cooked chicken
3. Add applesauce and stir until evenly mixed

Creamy Mushroom Turkey:

1 lb. ground turkey
1 can of Campbell's "98% fat free" cream of mushroom soup

1. Brown ground turkey in skillet
2. Drain cooked turkey
3. Add entire can of soup and stir until evenly mixed

Meat Stuffing:

1 lb. ground beef
1 lb. ground pork
1 cup chopped onions (frozen works well)
1 cup Ore-Ida frozen mashed potatoes
¼ tsp. poultry seasoning
¼ tsp. nutmeg
⅛ tsp. ground cloves
salt and pepper to taste

1. Combine beef, pork, spices, and onions in skillet and brown
2. Drain combination when done
3. Add mashed potatoes and stir until evenly mixed

After ten to twelve days of ground or pureed foods, you will progress to eating real, solid, ordinary food. No kidding! At times you can't wait to move back to real foods, but on the other hand, you can get pretty apprehensive about it because you get worried about the "sticking" you've heard about. Have no fear, we have all progressed through the stages and you will too. Just take a deep breath and get ready for it!

NOTES

8. Back To REAL Food (Stage 5)

Transitioning back to solid foods was very scary. For fourteen days, it was liquids or soft, mushy foods, which were pretty easy. I was always afraid that something would get "stuck" (and what won't go down must come back up...you get the picture)! But I was determined to keep on trying.

Rule of Three: Think of yourself as a very big baby. When babies are first introduced to solid foods, they try a new food every couple of days to make sure it's tolerated. You need to do the same thing, but you also have to do it a bite at a time. When you first start, take one bite of food, wait five minutes. If you're not feeling sick (nauseous) or the food doesn't feel like it's stuck, then take a second bite. Again, wait five minutes. Take a third bite (hence the "rule of three") and wait the five minutes one last time. If after that you're not experiencing any difficulties, then finish eating that food and check it off as something you've conquered. It's a long, slow process those first few weeks back on real food. But it will work and you'll eventually be eating all solid foods again.

The biggest change was how much more I wanted to enjoy really flavorful foods. Before my surgery, I was a very basic cook (just ask my family)! Dinner consisted of thawing out my meat of choice, adding a bottle of the "flavor of the day," baking for thirty minutes, and being done! But it gets tricky when you have to have no added sugars. There are a few "low carb" sauces out there, but they're hard to find.

One company that carries great items made with Splenda is Steel's Gourmet (www.steelsgourmet.com). They have all kinds of sauces, salad dressings, fruit spreads, dessert sauces, and even pie fillings.

They're not cheap, but if you're looking for something different, they've got it. Delmonte has a new organic tomato paste that is made without sugar (unlike regular paste). There are also canned fruits (pineapple, peaches, and pears) that are "no sugar added." Also, try some of the Campbell's 98 percent fat free soups to use in your cooking.

Organic products won't help too much as they are usually sweetened with "pure cane juice," and those kinds of sweeteners are just all natural versions of sugar. That will NOT work! South Beach Diet has some high protein bars that are made with Splenda which are good for snacks and meal substitutes.

Remember, take it slow and chew your food thoroughly. You need to realize that you are re-training your mind as well as your body how you eat, what you eat, and what your new portion sizes should be. **It's a gigantic task and deserves all the attention you can give it!** Keep track of your protein and liquid intake with the DTS (see forms in Appendices) and update it as you add new foods or find that you stop eating certain foods. Keep track of your daily medications and supplements by using one of those "day of the week" pill boxes. Life can be crazy, and by taking the worry out of remembering to do all that you have to do each day, you'll be a lot better off.

9.Supplements Galore

Multivitamin: You'll need to take an adult dose multivitamin every day for the rest of your life starting right after surgery. Try the One-A-Day Children's Multivitamin (Bugs Bunny, Scooby Doo, etc.). Any multivitamin will do, but if you've ever tasted the inside of an adult multivitamin, it's about the worst smelling and tasting thing on the planet! Stick with the kids' version (at least until you can swallow pills whole, which is two to three months after surgery).

Calcium: Starting one month after surgery and forever, you will need to take 1,200 milligrams a day of calcium. You can buy pills (Citrical or Caltrate) or try the chews (Viactiv—make sure to buy the sugar-free ones, which I found easily at Wal-Mart). The tricky part is that only five hundred mg. will be absorbed at a time. That means that you have to space the two doses at least four hours apart in order for them to have the full absorption. Again, keeping track on the DTS makes this easier so you don't miss a dose. Failure to consume enough calcium increases your risk of osteoporosis and bone fractures.

B12: One month after surgery and forever, you will take five hundred mcg. sublingual (under the tongue—it dissolves) every day. I did it for about one month and then gave up and decided to have a monthly B12 injection instead. Anything to reduce the number of pills to take in a day! Because your body no longer absorbs B12 as well as it did before GBS, you are at risk for anemia (which, left untreated, can lead to a whole host of problems you don't want to deal with).

Iron: After the first month, most patients are instructed to take 325 mg. of iron daily. The trouble with iron is that it reduces the effective absorption of all kinds of prescription and over-the-counter medications (including the calcium you have to take). Iron has to be separated from calcium by at least four hours. Personally, I take Synthroid (for my thyroid), which also has to be spaced by at least four hours from iron. So it becomes a tricky game like a jigsaw puzzle.

Make sure to check with your physician or pharmacist as to which medicines you're taking and make sure you don't need to do any spacing of your pills. Failure to take daily iron may result in anemia.

About two years out from my GBS, my iron was getting dangerously low—to the point where the doctor was talking about iron intravenous infusions. That didn't sound like anything I wanted to have to do, so I started researching other methods of getting iron into my system because the regular ferrous sulfate iron made me constipated and I couldn't take it (which is why my iron levels were dropping).

I found information on another kind of iron (iron bisglycinate) that is far more absorbable (45 percent compared to 3 percent), doesn't break down in the digestive tract, and won't cause stomach irritation or constipation. A company called Wellness Resources (www.wellnessresources.com) had a supplement called Blood Builder that contained this form of iron, so I bought it and gave it a try. After about one month on the pills, my iron was back up in the "normal" range and without the nasty side effects of the other iron pills.

Antacids: You will need to take Tums (also gives you calcium) daily or even a prescription such as Zantac or Prevacid. Your new pouch is so small that any additional acid can really do damage, so these products will most likely be taken daily for life. If you do start to experience heartburn or any other gastro-intestinal symptoms, you need to notify your doctor immediately for either a medication adjustment or further testing.

10.Back to Reality

Cookbooks: You don't need to buy special cookbooks with recipes just for GBS patients (unless you want to, that is)! You can buy any diabetic, Atkins, or South Beach cookbooks. They all use sugar substitutes and that's really the bottom line. You can also take most recipes and alter them yourself. As long as they are using regular white sugar (not molasses or brown sugar), then you can just substitute the white sugar the recipe calls for with Splenda (or Equal).

I did that with a recipe for sweet and sour sauce and was pleasantly surprised how little difference there was. The trick is to buy all kinds of fresh herbs and spices and try new things. When you eat such small portions, you will find that you want it to taste fantastic, not just average.

Going to parties: The safest thing to do about parties is to assume that there will not be any great foods there to help you achieve your daily protein target. Therefore, you have to plan on getting your protein in before the party or after you get home. Once there, see if there's anything with protein and nibble on that. You can usually find cheese or sometimes shrimp cocktail or something along those lines. Stay away from the high-fat chips and dips and obviously anything with sugar in it.

If the party is at someone's home (vs. a restaurant or function hall), bring your own beverage. All of my friends got used to me lugging around my sport bottle with my peach iced tea and said nothing (and in fact were very supportive)! When you get further along and can have a drink with alcohol in it, stick to wine (fewer calories and only natural sugars).

But if mixed drinks are more your thing, try the Baja Bob brand of mixers (www.bajabob.com). They make all kinds of cocktail mixes (martini, margarita, mojito, etc.) that use Splenda instead of sugar and are absolutely out of this world! I even have friends who have switched to it because they taste great but don't have all the calories, sugars, and carbs of the regular mixes. They're great for having a drink or two of something fun and trendy (say an apple martini) while staying within your new diet guidelines. However, don't plan on any of these for at least six to twelve months after GBS.

Eating out: One of the things that bothered me was all the people who said that after the GBS they couldn't go out to eat anymore. I thought that was such a shame because to me that's one of life's greatest joys. If you're going to a restaurant, make sure you pick something that's high in protein—in other words, don't go to Olive Garden and order a bowl of spaghetti! Order a chicken marsala dish instead. So you only eat a quarter of the food on the plate, who cares?! Wrap it up and take it home for the next day's lunch (and dinner again). Or leave it behind. You've spent more money over the years on diet programs that failed. At least with this expense you're getting food that tastes fabulous and you get to go out with friends and family and have fun.

Staying home and hiding in your house is silly. Get out there and enjoy your newly emerging physical self and have fun! If the waitress asks if something is wrong with your food, just say, "No, I'm just full, but I'd love to take it home" or "I'm dieting," which everyone understands. No big deal!

Eating at the cafeteria (at work): It's like anything else after GBS...you need to plan ahead. Think about what items they offer that are high in protein. There's usually tuna, chicken, or egg salad in the deli. Just ask for one scoop of the stuff, no bread. Or if there's a grilled chicken breast sandwich on the menu, buy it and then discard the "sandwich" portion of it and just eat the grilled chicken. If you can bring your own lunch, then obviously that's the way to go. But if you work at some of the bigger companies that frown on that, you'll have to figure out what the cafeteria (or local restaurant) can come up with.

There's no need to go into the details with the cafeteria/restaurant staff about why you need something different, just order what you want. Remember, you're paying for it—if you want to throw out your bread or not eat the potatoes that come with the item, that's your choice. It seems that everyone is on a diet of some kind or another these days, so no one really asks most of the time.

Eating on the go: Another thing to think about is buying easily portable foods. Items like individually wrapped cheese sticks (in the dairy aisle) were a great way to get my protein in if I had a day of errands and running around where I would not be able to sit for a meal. Oscar Mayer Lunchables also makes a great snack of crackers, lunch meat, and cheese (think mini-sandwiches with the crackers in place of bread). To this day I still have a half-dozen of them in the refrigerator at all times for whenever I have to run out of the house. Being prepared for unexpected situations is always a smart thing.

Illnesses: remember to keep sugar-free cough medicines on hand. The only problem is that they are fairly weak and if you get a really bad cough, they're not much help. One time I got a terrible cold that had me coughing so badly I was pulling muscles in my back and practically broke a rib as a result. I finally called my internist and he was able to call in a sugar-free prescription cough medicine that had codeine in it to quiet the cough so I could get some sleep.

Who knew they made such things in sugar free?! Because I didn't want to bother my doctor with a "stupid cough" and because I waited so long, I actually made myself worse. There's no shame in calling to see if there's something that can be done for you that is sugar free that the over-the-counter medicines just don't have. Because of the prevalence of diabetes, there are lots of sugar-free medicines available today.

Pain relievers: Due to the increased risk of bleeding and developing ulcers in your new smaller stomach, medicines containing ibuprofen (Advil, Motrin) and naproxen (Aleve) are no longer allowed. Make sure that you have acetaminophen products (Tylenol) on hand for all your aches and pains.

Exercise: Introducing exercise (even ten minutes a day) is vital to successful post-op health. Be honest with yourself about what you will and will not do. Don't go out and spend $1,000 on a yearly gym membership and then go twice and never again. Find a place that will let you pay by the month. Or invest in a few small hand weights and do simple exercises at home. If you need to be "guided" but can't afford a gym, try buying a workout video and use it at home. You can also hire a personal trainer to come and show you what exercises to do, and then do them on your own after that.

No exercise is effective if you don't do it.! Anything you find that will work for you is the right thing! You will develop certain "trouble areas": inner and outer thighs, buttocks, belly, and upper arms (triceps). These are the areas most affected by extra sagging skin and higher than normal fat deposits. There are many exercises that you can try to tone these, but at some point, it's just excess skin that is not going to go away. Some things may require plastic surgery to fix (see Chapter 13).

Support group: Make sure you find out when your program has a support group session and attend as often as your schedule allows. These groups are often made up of other patients at various stages of the GBS process, doctors, nurses, and a host of other guests. It helps to be able to talk to others who have been through GBS for advice and support. When things are tough, it's nice to know that you have understanding people to talk to who won't judge you or think your questions are silly or pointless. As you progress through the process, you then become one of the "teachers" and "supporters" for new patients, and that has its own benefits.

11.Unexpected Weight Loss Issues

There are so many "perks" to losing weight that I can't possibly mention them all. But let me mention some of the more exciting ones. There are the obvious ones like the fact that when you go on an airplane you don't have to ask for the seatbelt extender or worry that you'll "ooze" over that imaginary line and invade the space of the person sitting next to you with your larger than normal self. You can go to amusement parks again and actually get buckled into the big roller coasters (or fit into the teacups if that's more your speed)! When you go to a family cookout, you can actually sit in one of those stackable plastic chairs and not have to spend the entire four hours acting like you enjoy standing (or sitting on the ground).

Disappearing aches: Things that used to hurt and ache don't seem to do that anymore. The feet, knees, ankles, back, or whatever area the weight was harming seems to have simply stopped hurting (or hurts a lot less).

Reduction in medicines: If you were on medications for diabetes, high blood pressure, and some of the other problems affected by obesity, lots of times your medications are reduced or even stopped altogether. It is a great feeling to know that your body is regulating itself again without medication making it work. You are adding healthy years to your life.

Changing sizes: All your sizes keep dropping from shoes, to rings, to clothes. The clothing thing can be annoying at times because you have to keep buying new clothes every four to six weeks, which can become expensive (especially if you have a high-powered job that requires real suits and not just jeans or sweats). If at all possible, choose things with drawstring or elastic waists so that it will last you several sizes. Another good thing to invest in is a basic belt.

After a while, it becomes exhilarating to go shopping for new clothes. Once you get over the fact that you can no longer shop at that plus size or big men's store, the choices of great clothes that are available for you to wear become unbelievable. The colors and fabrics that they use in "regular" size clothing are so much more impressive. And for me, who is all of five feet two inches tall, I was able to shop in the petite departments again and actually get things that I didn't have to turn the cuffs up on or take to the tailors to be shortened. Wow!

Adjustments: One of the little things that I didn't expect was the fact that I kept adjusting the seat in my car forward every few weeks. As I had gotten bigger over the years, I kept adjusting it farther and farther back so the steering wheel didn't dig into my stomach, but I never realized that I was doing that. And then when I lost nine inches around my hips, it made sense that I'd have to move my seat closer because my feet were too far from the pedals. Not a big thing, but it just goes to show how many accommodations we have to make over the years that we don't even realize.

Arctic zone: Another strange "side effect" of the GBS was that once I had lost about sixty pounds, I found that I was always cold. Now, you might be saying, well, I get cold easily now. But you see, for me, I was always too warm. My husband used to call me his "personal heater" because if he got cold in the middle of the night he could roll over and I'd be nice and warm. But I got to the point where I was taking hot showers at ten p.m. because I just couldn't warm up despite socks and sweatshirts, etc.! After a while (it's different with everyone), this lessens. But most of my friends in support group say that even two years out they're still colder than they ever were before. Guess it's true that fat is a great insulator because it really kept me warm.

Reactions of others: The biggest thing that you start to notice (other than your baggy clothes) is the reactions of other people about your weight loss. I was very fortunate that every single person I came into contact with (even people I barely knew) was happy for me and told me how great I looked and to keep up the good work. The only problem for me was learning to accept a compliment on my physical appearance. For twenty years (or more), no one had done that and in the beginning it was hard to take. Now, I love it!

Other GBS patients have different experiences that aren't so great. Sometimes spouses and family members are threatened by this new, thinner person and try to sabotage their success by offering them treats and trying to get them to eat more. Sometimes people will suddenly take notice of you now that you're thin and start being nice to you when they weren't interested in you when you were obese. As if somehow now that you are thinner you are more "worthy" of their association.

There is also a higher than average divorce rate after GBS. As a patient loses weight, his or her self-esteem increases. GBS can make good marriages better and bad marriages worse. Sometimes GBS patients were in abusive relationships and once they gained more self-confidence they realized that they weren't willing to allow the situation to continue. Others feel that they want something more or better than before. Sometimes the non-GBS spouse has a need to be the "more attractive" one and can't handle the competition.

All of these situations can be extremely hard to deal with and lead to feelings of confusion and anger. If you experience these kinds of issues, you should seek help by talking to a therapist or psychiatrist. Your weight center or insurance company should be able to suggest some professionals you could contact. You can also bring up these issues at your support group.

NOTES

12.New Treats

Most of us are used to rewarding ourselves with "treats" such as cookies, cakes, pies, etc. In your new life after GBS, you need to find ways of rewarding yourself in other ways. For me, my first reward was after I lost fifty pounds. I decided to get my hair cut and professionally colored (which I had never done). It was the best $100 I had spent in twenty years! It gave me a real lift and started people noticing me and all that I had lost.

It was great to hear my best friend's husband say, "Wow, you're becoming a real babe!" In my entire adult life, no one had ever said anything so nice to me.

Go to your local department store and have them do your makeup an hour or so before you meet your husband for dinner. It won't cost you a thing and you'll look and feel great. I also found that after losing so much weight, I had aches and knots in my body that I hadn't been aware of, so I got a massage at a local spa and felt so much looser and better.

If you enjoy sports, treat yourself to tickets to a ball game or to a session of paint ball or laser tag. There has to be something you have always wanted to do or wished your size didn't prevent you from doing. Start putting some time and energy into your newly emerging thinner self. You've avoided paying attention to that person for too long—you're worth it!

Clothes shopping, depending on your budget, can be a challenge. Unless you're rolling in dough, you should plan on buying a few basic items that mix and match (think "Garanimals" for grown-ups)! All you really need is two pairs of pants (or skirts) and four tops that will go with both pairs of pants (or skirts). I was able to get away with jeans, but I still bought two pairs and rotated them. You're also going to have to buy new undergarments and even shoes. So buy wisely and remember that every month or so you'll have to buy the next smaller size. And for goodness sakes, buy a belt and tuck in your shirt!

It's amazing, but as I dropped the weight, I never wanted to wear big, baggy clothes anymore. The other thing to think about is that no one really cares what you wear as long as it's appropriate for the occasion (work, cookout, etc.). So save your money for the new wardrobe you will buy when you have reached your goal weight and just "make do" in the meantime. Less is definitely more in this case. And make sure to donate your old clothes and take that tax deduction. Your "loss" is definitely someone else's gain.

Remember that photo I told you to take in a bathing suit?! Well, at about five or six months after the GBS, take it out again and really look at it. You'll see what I was talking about. Take another picture in a new bathing suit at six months and again at one year (and so on). This is going to be the set of photos you will want to keep to always remind you of how far you've come and that you never want to go back again.

Now that I eat such small meals, I want them to be really full of flavor. As a result, I have gotten hooked on watching the Food Network. When I first started doing it, my family thought I was nuts and I think they were a little worried that I was longing for food again, but I wasn't. I just love to watch their shows and get ideas for recipes I can make that are new and different for me. Evidently, I'm not the only one because most of my support group friends have also become fans of the network.

The thing that I found the most unexpected as my body was shrinking was the feeling of power I now felt inside. My life was still my crazy and chaotic life. My kids were just as out of control at times, my husband's job was just as all-consuming, my bills still needed to be paid, and my house still needed to be taken care of. But in the midst of it all, I felt an inner peace that made dealing with the craziness of life so much easier.

I felt such a huge sense of accomplishment for having made a good decision (to have the GBS) and for giving 400 percent effort every day to make it work. I felt that I had been able to take control of my obesity instead of it always being in control of me. I was no longer its victim and that made me feel like I could do anything I set my mind to. If I could make the great, big scary journey through GBS and beyond, then I could deal with anything life had to throw my way. The day in and day out stresses of my life haven't changed, but I have changed and become a more fulfilled, stronger, and happier person (inside and out) and that has been the most thrilling "perk" to losing the weight!

NOTES

13.Plastic Surgery & Beyond

The only unfortunate outcome of GBS is the excess skin that you're left with after losing all the weight (and even before you reach your goal). The first one that struck me was what I lovingly refer to as my "bat wings." That's the saggy skin under your upper arms that flaps when you shake your arms (like a bat flying...). I asked my doctor if there were any exercises I could do to help shrink that and she said that she hated to disappoint me, but I could work out for eight hours a day and not shrink that skin. The only way it leaves is under a plastic surgeon's knife.

There are, of course, other areas that develop these big baggy, saggy pieces of skin that are no longer filled with fat but have nowhere to go because you stretched them out. Most common are the belly, the inner and outer thighs, and the face and/or neck. For women there are also the breasts that have now fallen way south of where they should be (and if you've had children or breastfed, you're really toast)! If you can afford it, all of these issues can be fixed with plastic surgery. But it's not cheap or painless. It should also not be done for at least one and a half to two years after your GBS.

One suggestion is that you take the money you used to spend on food (going out to dinner, desserts, etc.) that you can't have any more and put it in a special "plastic surgery fund" so that at the end of the two years, you might actually be able to afford some of the procedures you need. Think about it...if you put $50 away each week for two years, you'd have $5,200 to pay for plastic surgery (and if you put it in an interest bearing account, it'd be even more)!

That won't get everything fixed, but it would most likely take care of at least your biggest problem area. Just understand that it's part of the process and that the reason you did the GBS was to make yourself healthier and to enjoy a long life. Some of the skin might shrink back, but if it doesn't you either deal with it surgically or stoically, whichever works. Either way you are no longer obese and a few flaps of excess skin are a lot easier to deal with physically than all that you were dealing with before.

If you are going to go the plastic surgery route, start planning ahead. There's a "tummy tuck" to remove the very large extra flap of skin on your middle that for some people hangs so far down that it makes daily living a challenge, to say the least. Then there are the inner and outer thighs that are bulging and covered in extra saggy skin. Don't forget my personal favorite, the "bat wings" (the underside of the upper arms that waves when you wave). Let's not forget the breasts (mostly for women, but sometimes for men too). When you lose one hundred-plus pounds, you lose it in your bust too! What you have left after it's all said and done is either not much, way south of where it should be, or both.

There's also a butt lift where the excess skin and fat is removed and they give you a nice new, shapely butt. Each of these procedures costs anywhere from $3,000 to $10,000. Some procedures may be able to be done together, which will save you money on hospital and anesthesia costs (surgeon's fees don't diminish), but most likely you will need to have several separate surgeries, depending on what you want to "fix."

Make sure you choose a plastic surgeon who is familiar with the issues of patients who have lost extreme amounts of weight. Consider asking your GBS surgeon for a recommendation. Be open and honest about your finances as well as your wants and needs from a surgical standpoint.

If you think insurance will pay for any of this, think again! A few insurance companies will pay for a simple panniculectomy, which is just the removal of the skin apron on your mid-section. They will not pay for any body contouring (liposuction) or abdominal muscle tightening (abdominoplasty).

They also have a list of criteria that you must meet in order for the procedure to be covered. This usually consists of documentation of rashes, dermatological treatment, and prescriptions for antibiotics (oral and topical). Before you even go for a surgical consult, I recommend you find out what hoops your insurance company wants you to jump through before they pay. And then be prepared for them to deny payment! Basically, if they paid for the GBS, they figure anything else is cosmetic and not covered. So know that going into this and be prepared accordingly.

I decided to have the abdominoplasty/panniculectomy about eighteen months after my GBS. It was by far the most painful recovery of any surgery I had ever had. When they tighten all those abdominal muscles with those deep stitches, you basically have no use of those muscles for six to eight weeks. It was amazing how many things we do that use our abdominal muscles. Something as simple as coughing or closing a dresser drawer became impossible. It took a good eight weeks before I really felt that I had full use of those muscles.

Two years after my GBS, I then had the inner and outer thigh lifts done. The recovery from that surgery was much less painful, but presented its own set of difficulties. Make sure to ask your surgeon about any post-op needs you will have. There's nothing worse than getting home from the hospital, incapacitated with stitches and big incisions, only to find out that you need a certain support undergarment (like Spanx)! And with you not in any physical condition to get to the store, let alone try these things on! Best to ask LOTS of question before your surgery to be prepared and get any specialty shopping done beforehand.

NOTES

14.Then There's You

Well, my book is done! I hope you found some useful information and tips on how to help you through your own surgery. I also hope I was able to help you gain a better understanding of the day-to-day struggles you may find along the way to a new you.

I encourage you to contact me and let me know how you're doing. Remember, I'm not a physician, nutritionist, or psychiatrist, but I am a survivor. There is no foolish question except the one you don't ask. I can be reached by:

e-mail: lori@readysetshrink.com

snail mail: Lori Ferrante, P.O. Box 870191, Milton, MA 02187

website: www.readysetshrink.com

The journey was not always trouble-free, but I am glad that I made the choice I did. I am a much healthier person because of it. Good luck on your own journey and remember that with proper planning and a lot of perseverance, YOU CAN DO IT! I applaud you and your decision and look forward to hearing from you!

Websites you may find useful:

www.bajabob.com
www.campbells.com
www.chobani.com
www.crystallight.com
www.delmonte.com

www.fageusa.com
www.motts.com
www.obesityhelp.com
www.splenda.com
www.steelsgourmet.com
www.traderjoes.com
www.veryfine.com
www.vitaminshoppe.com
www.wellnessresources.com

Appendix 1 – Pre-Surgery Shopping List

Items To Be Purchased	Quantity Needed	✓ When Done
Sugar-free protein shakes	2-3 cases	
Sugar-free Jell-O cups	2 packages of 6	
Broth (chicken or beef)	1 container	
Sugar-free popsicles	1 box	
Diet/100% juice (apple, cranberry, etc.)	2 bottles	
Fage 0% yogurt (or similar)	6 containers	
GladWare mini rounds	2-3 containers of 8	
Food scale	1	
Small food processor/chopper	1	
Pill crusher	1	
Flavored waters (Fruit$_2$O or similar)	24 bottles	
Individual sugar-free powdered drink mixes (Crystal Light or similar)	2 boxes	
Non-stick gauze pads – large	2 boxes	
First aid tape	2 rolls	
Sugar-free children's chewable multivitamin	1 bottle	
Sugar-free calcium (Viactiv, Caltrate, etc.)	1 package	
Sugar-free Tums	1 bottle	
Tylenol "Go Tabs"	1 package	
Sugar-free cough syrup	1 bottle	
MedicAlert emblem	1	

Appendix 2 – Body Measurements

	Pre-Op	6 wks.	2 mths.	3 mths.	4 mths.	5 mths.	6 mths.
Weight							
Wrist							
Forearm							
Upper Arm							
Neck							
Bust							
Waist							
Hips							
Thigh							
Calf							
Ankle							
Ring Size							
Shoe Size							

Appendix 3 – Daily Tracking Sheet (Stage 3)

Item	SUN	MON	TUE	WED	THU	FRI	SAT
MEDICINES/SUPPLEMENTS:							
Multivitamin							
Calcium							
Iron							
B12							
Antacid							
PROTEINS: (4 oz. servings)							
PROTEIN (70g. = target)							
LIQUIDS:							
LIQUIDS (32oz. = min.)							

Appendix 4 – Daily Tracking Sheet (Stage 4)

Item	SUN	MON	TUE	WED	THU	FRI	SAT
MEDICINES/SUPPLEMENTS:							
PROTEIN: (4 oz. servings of each)							
PROTEIN GRAMS (70 = target)							
LIQUIDS: (16 oz. bottles)							
LIQUID OUNCES (32 = minimum)							

Appendix 5 – Daily Tracking Sheet (Stage 5)

	SUN	MON	TUE	WED	THU	FRI	SAT
MEDICINES/SUPPLEMENTS:							
PROTEIN: (4 oz. servings of each)							
PROTEIN GRAMS (70 = target)							
LIQUIDS:							
LIQUID OUNCES (32= minimum)							

Appendix 6 – Sugars

Acceptable:

aspartame
Equal
fructose
lactose
Nutra-Sweet
saccharin
Splenda
sucralose

Not Acceptable:

brown sugar
cane sugar (pure/organic)
confectioner's sugar
corn syrup
high-fructose corn syrup
honey
maple syrup
molasses
sucrose
sugar
turbinado sugar

Appendix 7 – Protein Sources

Food	Serving Size	Protein Grams Per Serving
Beans (dried or cooked)	½ cup	6-9
Beef (ground or whole)	1 ounce	7
Cheese (reduced fat or fat-free)	1 ounce	5-6
Chicken (ground or whole)	1 ounce	8
Cold cuts (turkey, etc.)	1 slice	7
Cottage cheese	¼ cup	6
Egg (salad, scrambled, etc.)	each	7
Fage 0% yogurt	5.3 ounces	13
Fish (cod, salmon, tuna, etc.)	1 ounce	7
Fruit	½ cup/1 small	1
Milk (fat-free, lactaid, soy)	½ cup	4-5
Nuts	½ cup	8
Nut butters (creamy or chunky)	1 tbsp.	4
Oatmeal	½ cup	5
Pork (ground or whole)	1 ounce	7
Protein shake	½ cup	7-12
Shellfish (shrimp, lobster, etc.)	1 ounce	7
Soups	½ cup	2-4
Tofu	1 ounce	2
Turkey (ground or whole)	1 ounce	7
Vegetables (raw, cooked, frozen, canned)	½ cup	2
Vegetables (leafy, loose packed)	1 cup	2